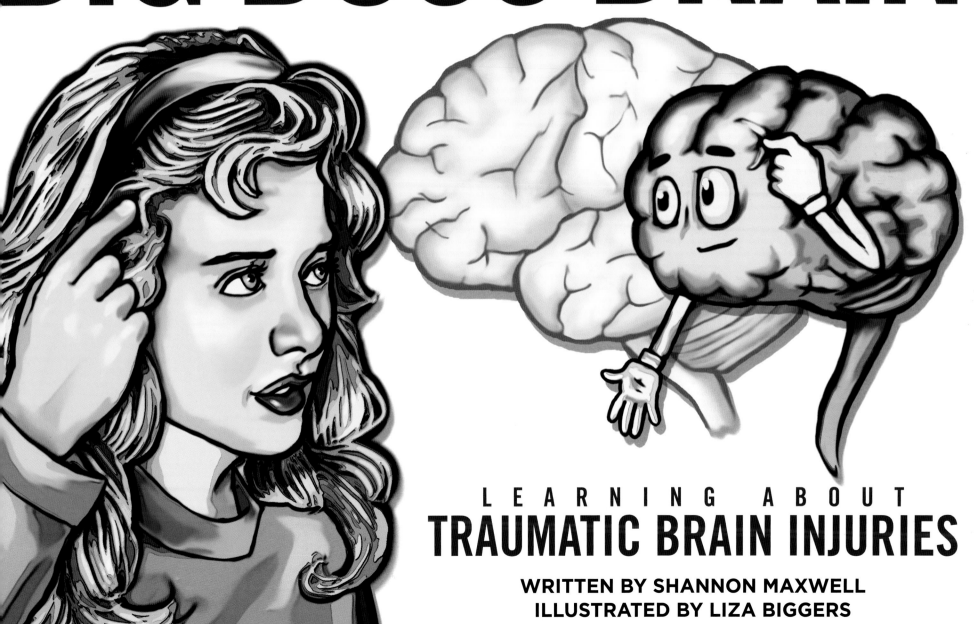

BIG BOSS BRAIN

LEARNING ABOUT
TRAUMATIC BRAIN INJURIES

WRITTEN BY SHANNON MAXWELL
ILLUSTRATED BY LIZA BIGGERS

ISBN 978-1-61751-006-9

Text copyright© 2012 by Shannon Maxwell
Illustrations copyright© 2012 by Liza Biggers.
All rights reserved.

Published by 4th Division Press
an imprint of E L Kurdyla Publishing LLC

LCCN: 2012904204

Printed in South Korea on acid-free paper

First Printing, 2012

Author's Dedication

This book is dedicated to my children, Alexis, Eric, and Cassidy, and all those children with a family member recovering from a traumatic brain injury. Thank you for the joy and energy you bring to the household and for your unconditional love throughout the healing process.

Believe that time heals wounds.

Find **hope** in the newness and possibilities each day brings.

Seize the new adventures and activities with your mom or dad.

Always **remember** to enjoy being a child.

Know that the love you share is the strongest weapon against all hurt and the brightest beam of light to guide you to new levels of happiness.

Illustrator's Dedication

This book is dedicated to my wonderful husband, Charlie, who is always willing to model for reference and is constantly my support through late nights of illustrating.

Letter to the Adults

According to the Centers for Disease Control and Prevention, "recent data shows that, on average, approximately 1.7 million people sustain a traumatic brain injury (TBI) annually." Ranging from "mild" to "severe" and at all ages and walks of life, the often-invisible effects are difficult for adults to fully comprehend, more so for children who are discovering the world around them. *Big Boss Brain* was created and written to help children better understand what may be happening to a loved one after brain injury and find hope in the possibilities of a changed but love-filled life together. Due to the severity of some individuals' injuries, the level of interaction between children and their loved ones compared to that depicted in the book may vary; however, this book seeks to instill acceptance so that in large or small ways, children can continue to find their family member a part of their lives.

While the story is largely based on our family's experiences, those of many of the TBI families we have encountered along the way are interwoven to create a fuller picture of the possible effects. We hope that this book will foster rich, positive conversations with your children and each other. Take comfort in knowing you are not alone, and believe in the possibilities!

—Shannon

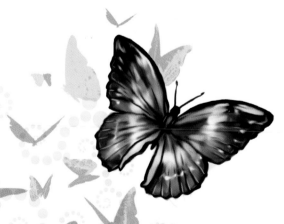

The butterfly is a symbol of **HOPE**. Throughout the story there are butterflies—some hidden, some not. Look and see if you can find them all. Clues are found on page 39.

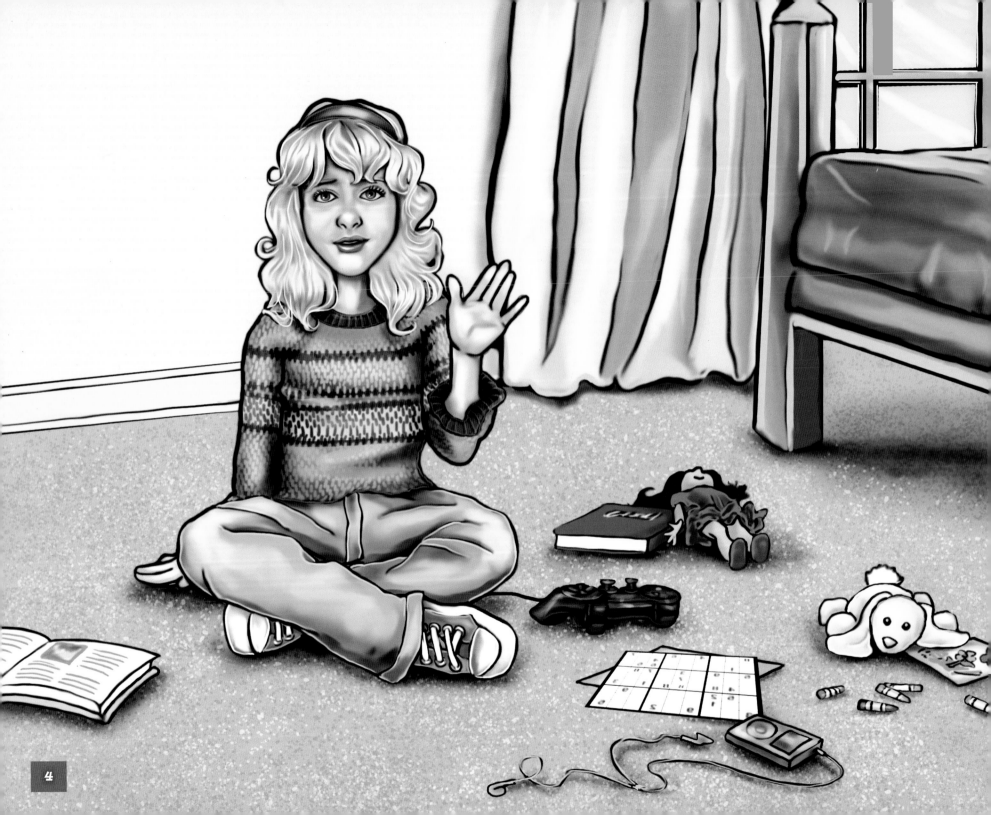

Hi! My name is Cassidy, and I have a ***traumatic brain injury***—TBI for short. You wouldn't know it by looking at or talking to me. This injury is often called an "invisible" injury. You can't always see it. It's deep inside my head. Think of when you have a stomachache. You can't see your stomachache, and neither can others, but it's there.

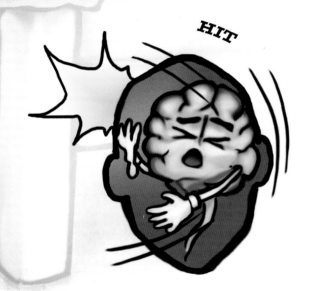
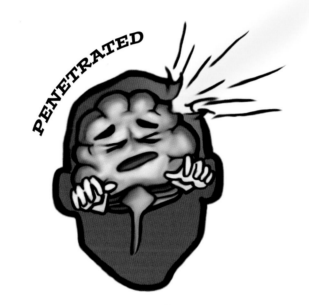
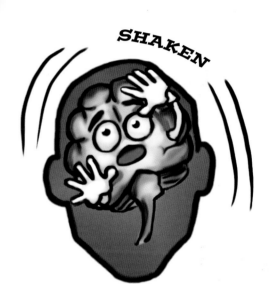

A TBI happens when something ***hits*** a person's head with a lot of power, something ***penetrates*** (breaks) through the skull, or a strong force ***shakes*** the head very fast, so that the soft brain bounces against the inside of the skull. It sounds scary, and it can be, but with time people can improve.

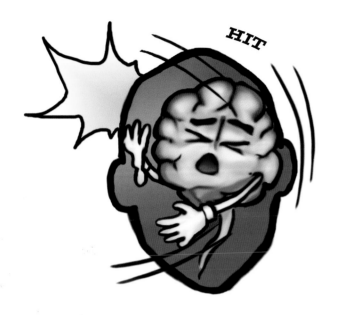

When I was two, my mom and I were in a terrible car crash. I was rushed to the hospital. Nurses and doctors helped me to get better. I'm almost ten now. Like other children my age, I read and run and play with friends. But I still have a reminder of my **_TBI_**.

On the right side of my head, hidden by my hair, I have a scar shaped like a "C." This is where the doctor operated. He fixed part of my hard, boney skull that pushed in on my soft brain when my head **_hit_** the car door. Since my name starts with a "C," I think this is pretty special. It makes me a unique, one-of-a-kind, special kid. It is also something I have in common with my daddy.

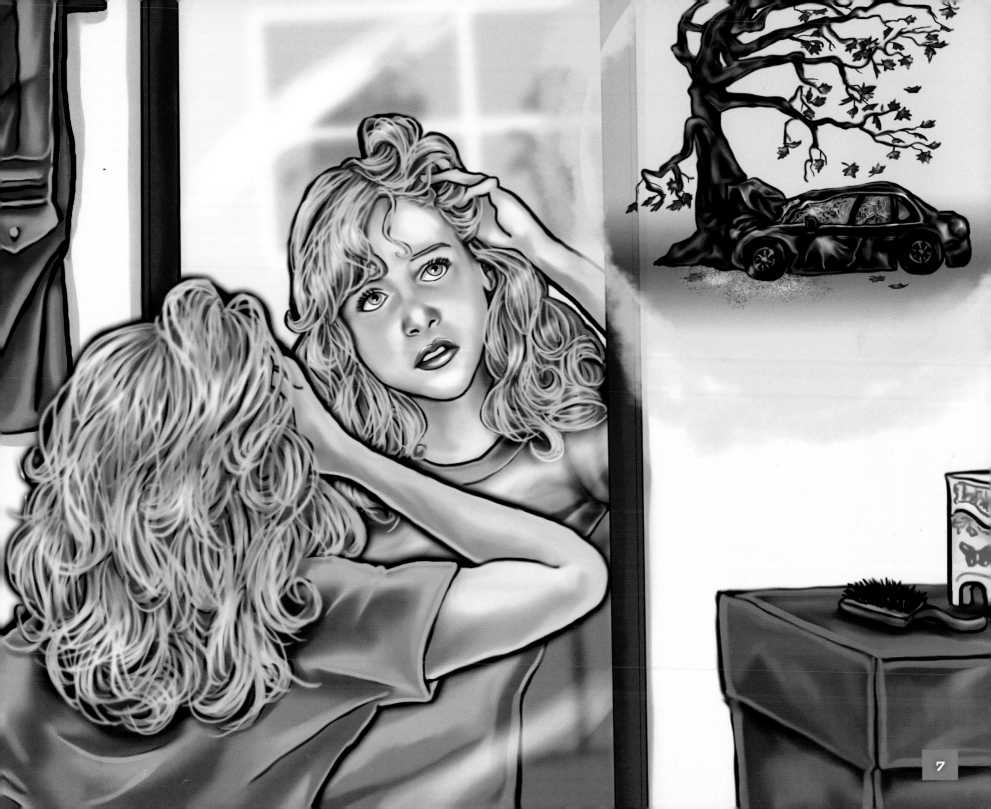

7

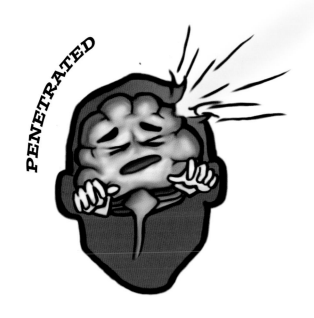
PENETRATED

You see, Daddy has a scar on his head, too. His scar is shaped like a big question mark. Daddy has a "penetrating TBI." One day, a mortar (a kind of bomb) exploded near him. Two little pieces of the metal bomb broke through the left side of his hard, boney skull and got into his soft brain.

Just like me, Daddy was rushed to a hospital. A doctor called a *neurosurgeon* fixed places in his brain that were bleeding. The doctor also took out a piece of Daddy's skull bone (about the size of a lemon). He closed the skin with big staples. This way, Daddy's swelling brain would not push against his hard, boney skull and be hurt more.

It left Daddy with a soft spot, so he had to wear a helmet to protect his brain. Daddy's head looked out of shape. After the swelling stopped, the doctors replaced the skull bone, and he looked like himself again.

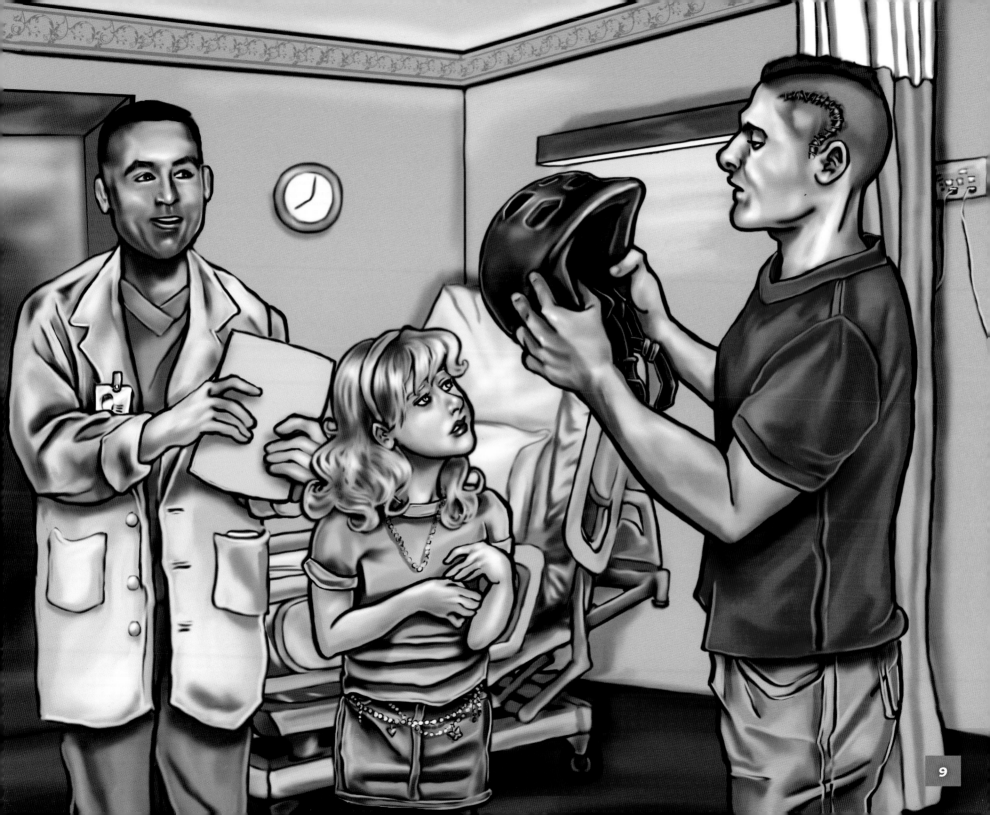

Since Daddy has short hair, I can see his scar every day. At bedtime, I rub it and give it a big kiss. Daddy's scar is *special*, too. It is a reminder that his life was saved when he was injured, helping others in a far-away place. He was there helping people to have freedom just like we do in America.

Sometimes Daddy will show me pictures of friends he met in the hospital. His friend Sam does not have a scar like Daddy and me. He has a "closed head TBI." Sam was hurt in a football game when he was tackled.

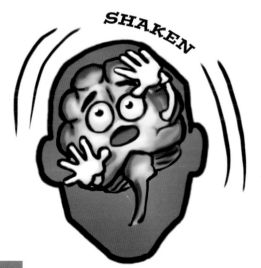

SHAKEN

The force **shook** Sam's brain against the inside of his hard skull. His body went to sleep for 16 days. Doctors call this type of sleep a **coma**. It's the body's way of sending all its healing energy to the brain. In Daddy's case, the doctors had to help his body sleep with medicines. That way, it could focus healing energy on his brain and not other parts of his body.

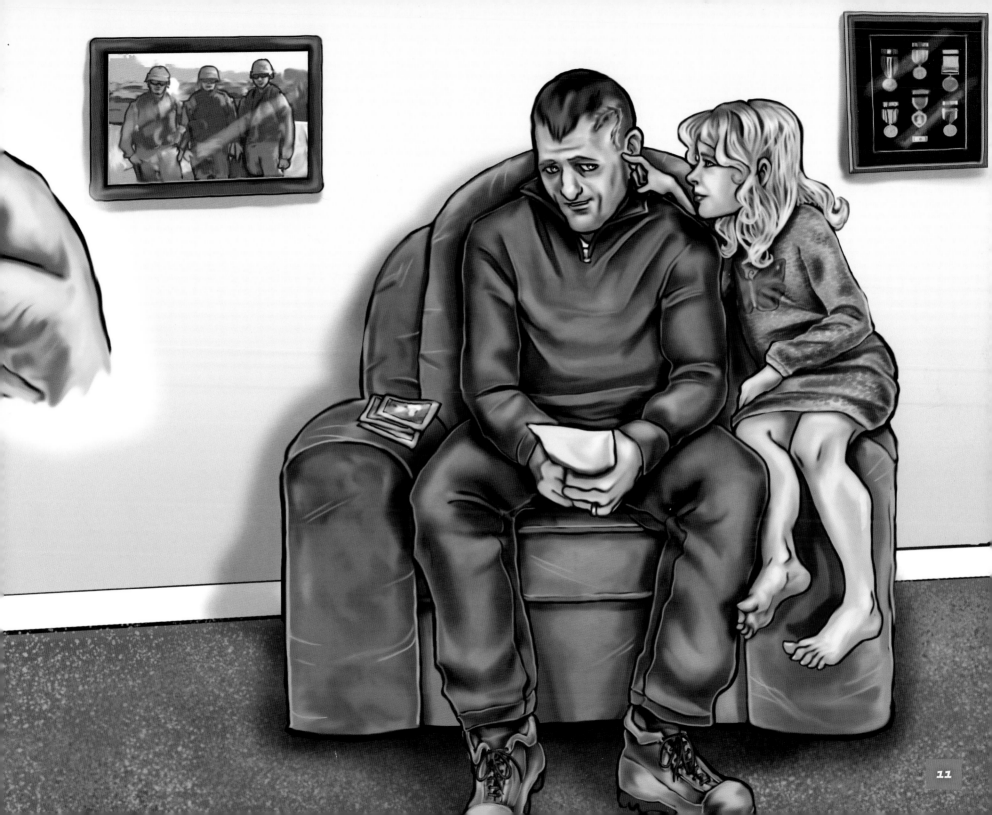

Every brain and every TBI and recovery is *different*. When I got hurt, I did not go into a coma like Sam and Daddy. After a couple of weeks, I was able to walk and go home from the hospital. It took Daddy and Sam months to get well enough to come home. When Daddy came out of his coma, at first he couldn't move the right side of his body or speak. He could only nod or shake his head to answer questions. He had to be pushed around in a wheelchair. Many different *therapists* helped Daddy relearn to talk, walk, and do everyday things. Calling the therapists SLPs, OTs, and PTs makes talking about TBI a lot easier!

"m...m...Medals... no...no... Med-i-cine"

Medicine

SLP

Speech Language Pathologists (SLPs) used picture cards and sticky note labels to help him remember words for many things.

Occupational Therapists (OTs) worked

with Daddy's fingers and hands. With time, his hand could grasp the spoon and lift it to his mouth.

OT

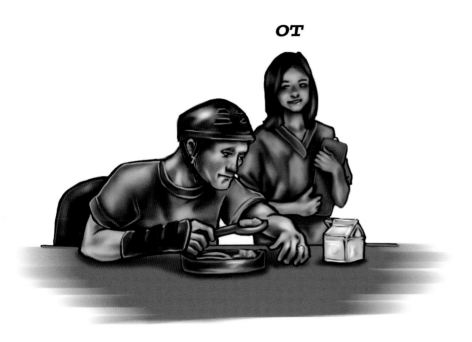

PT

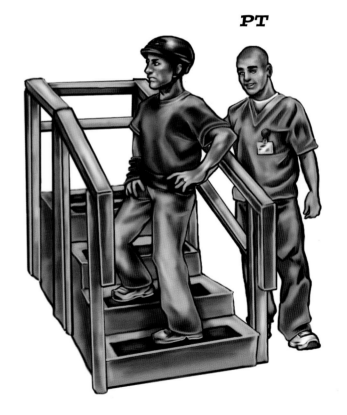

Physical Therapists (PTs) trained his

muscles and taught him exercises to help his brain remember how to move his legs.

13

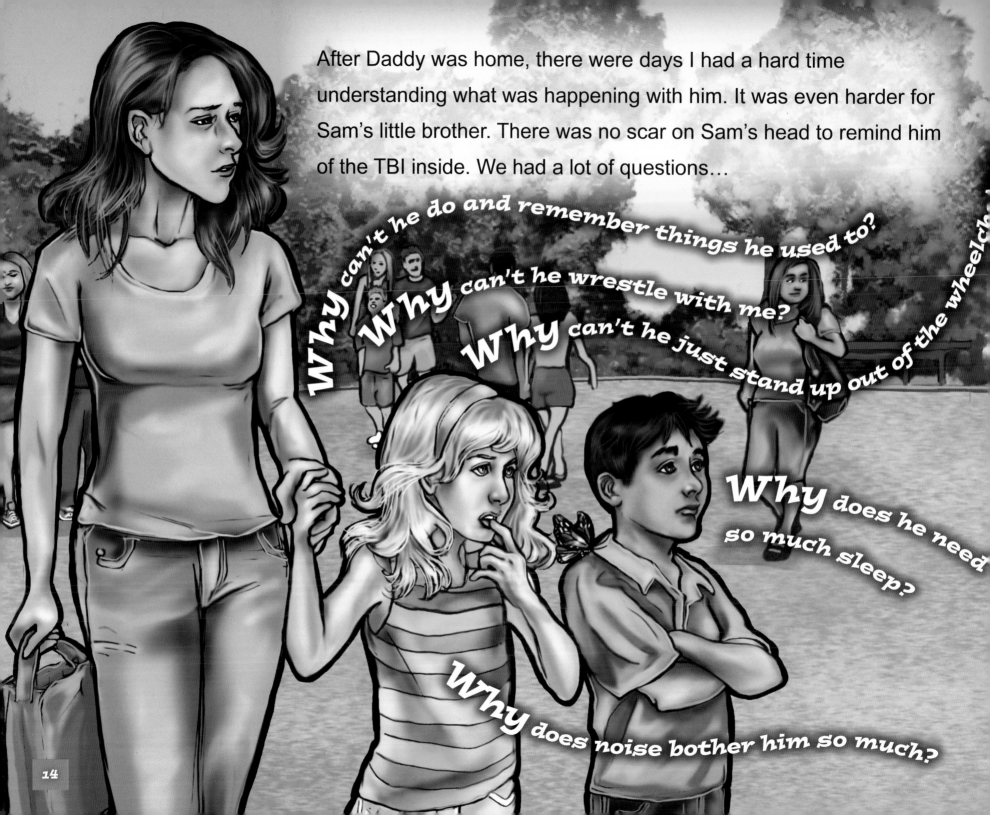

After Daddy was home, there were days I had a hard time understanding what was happening with him. It was even harder for Sam's little brother. There was no scar on Sam's head to remind him of the TBI inside. We had a lot of questions…

Why can't he do and remember things he used to?

Why can't he wrestle with me?

Why can't he just stand up out of the wheelchair?

Why does he need so much sleep?

Why does noise bother him so much?

14

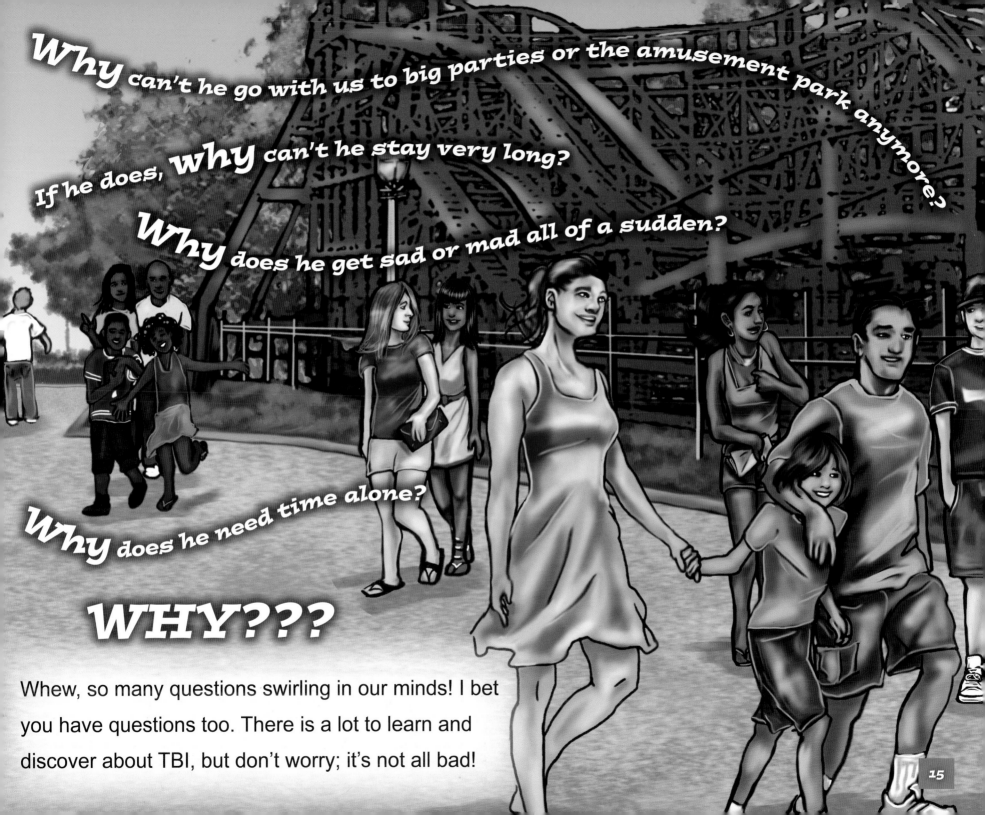

Why can't he go with us to big parties or the amusement park anymore?

If he does, why can't he stay very long?

Why does he get sad or mad all of a sudden?

Why does he need time alone?

WHY???

Whew, so many questions swirling in our minds! I bet you have questions too. There is a lot to learn and discover about TBI, but don't worry; it's not all bad!

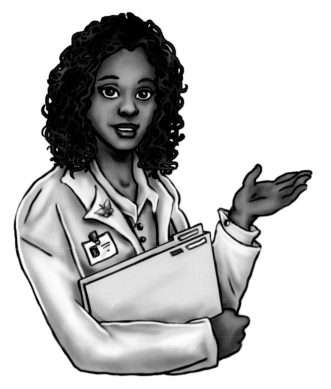

Daddy's case worker explained to me that Daddy's brain is the **"Big Boss"** of his body. Big Boss Brain tells different parts of the body what to do and how to do it, from breathing to moving a toe. Big Boss Brain even controls our ability to remember people, places, instructions, experiences, and *emotions*.

To see the parts of Big Boss Brain and what they do, turn to page 40.

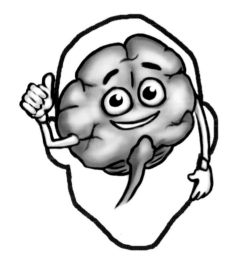

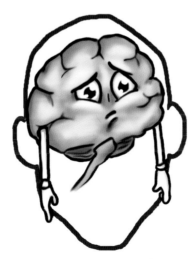

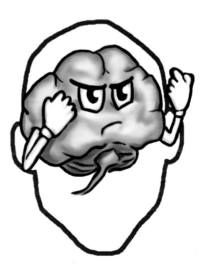

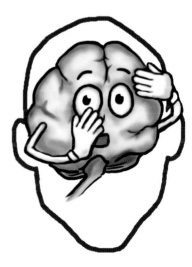

HAPPY   **SAD**   **ANGRY**   **SCARED**

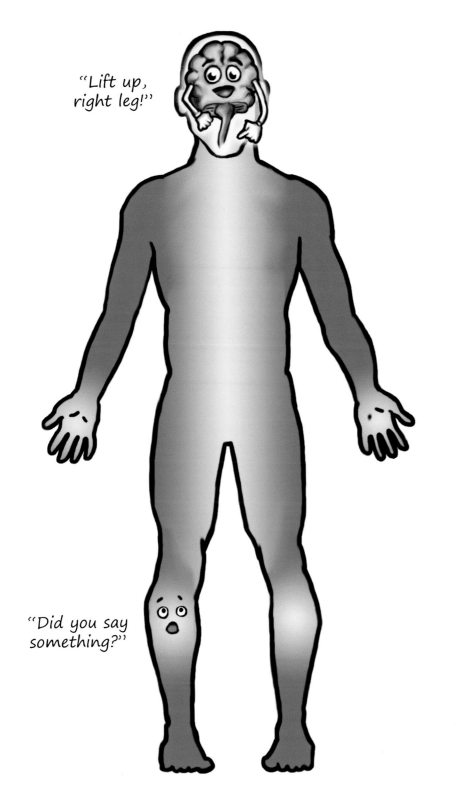

When part of the brain is hurt, things we do can change.

So when I wondered why Daddy couldn't wrestle with me or get out of his wheelchair, it was not that he didn't want to do those things. The reason was that the signals from Daddy's **Big Boss Brain** to his right arm and leg were broken. Big Boss Brain said, "Lift up right leg;" but his right leg was not getting the message.

Daddy's injuries were all on his left side, though. So why didn't his right side work? How confusing!

I found out that the left side of **Big Boss Brain** controls the right side of the body. The right side of Big Boss Brain controls the left side of the body. With lots of time and practice, Daddy began to move his right leg and arm. He worked hard with the therapists to make his right leg and arm stronger and to remind Big Boss Brain to focus on them.

It is important to know that sometimes, even with practice and hard work, Big Boss Brain is not able to get a signal working. Other times, it may not be able to make the signal strong enough to make things move like they used to. Daddy can walk now, but he has a limp. He can lift his right arm, but smaller movements like moving game pieces or cutting his meat are hard.

Daddy uses a special adaptive tool called a "rocker knife" to help him cut his meat now and a big calendar to remember events. The way he gives me big bear hugs has changed, too. With a lot of effort, Daddy can rest his right arm on my shoulder, but his hug is more with his left hand. It's different, but I know he still **loves** me.

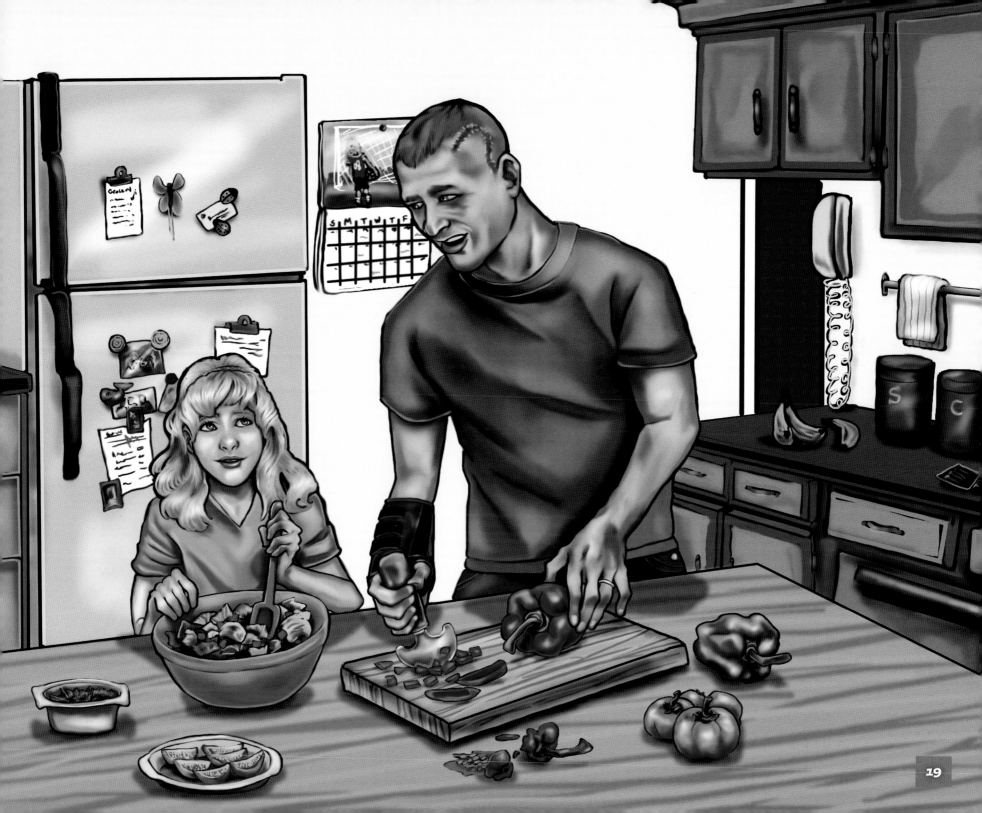

My friends Jake and Grace are also learning how different life can be after brain injury. Their parents still need their wheelchairs to get around. Their Big Boss Brains cannot tell their legs to stand up for long or, sometimes, at all.

Jake's dad's wheelchair has electric controls that can raise him up to a standing position. Jake says it makes his dad look a little like a robot. Pretty cool! The coolest part is that, even though his dad can't walk, his chair still lets him go to places with the family and play with Jake. Jake skates and races his dad down the sidewalk.

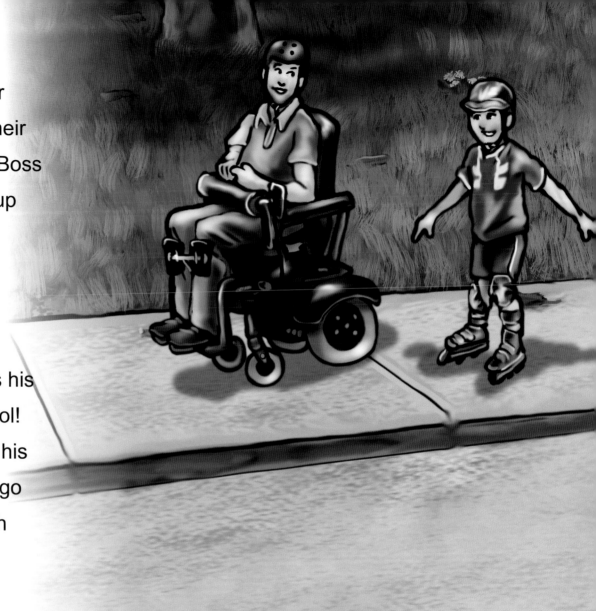

Grace's mom has a special bike that she and Grace's grandpa can ride together. Grace rides her bike alongside. Grace's mom has an *anoxic brain injury* from a motorcycle accident. "Anoxic" means her brain did not get enough oxygen for a long time. The brain uses oxygen as a source of energy. Without it, areas of her brain were damaged. My friends and I are learning that many changes come with TBI. We are also discovering new possibilities and ways to spend time together. You will too!

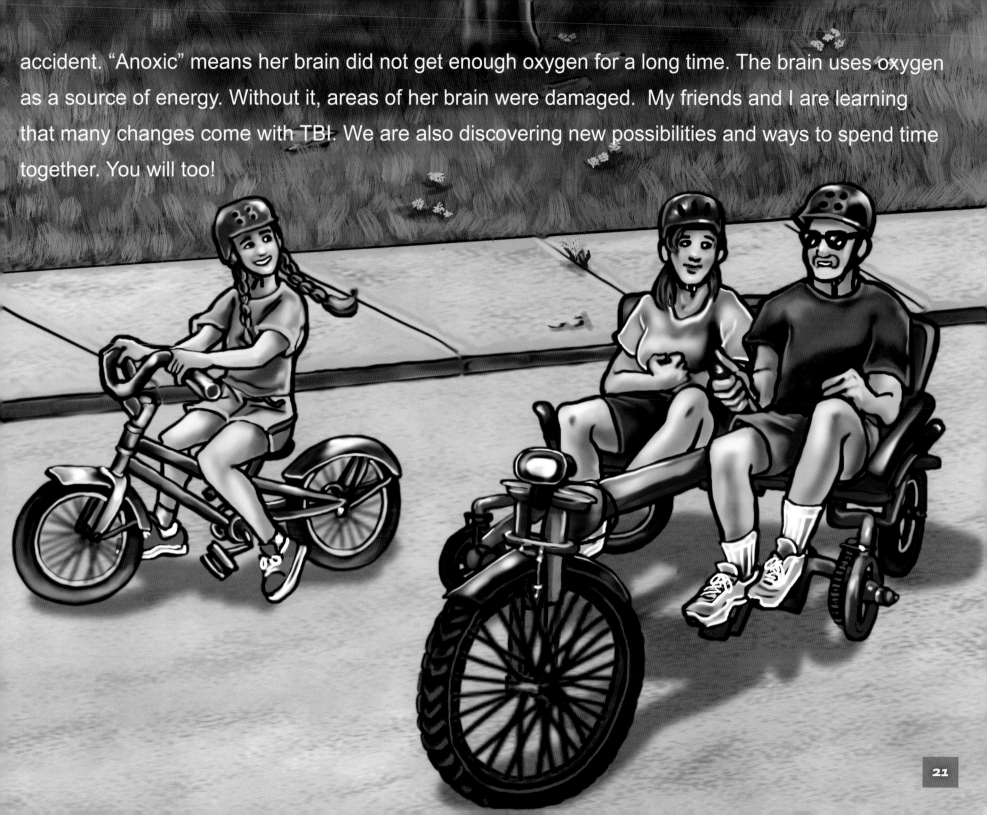

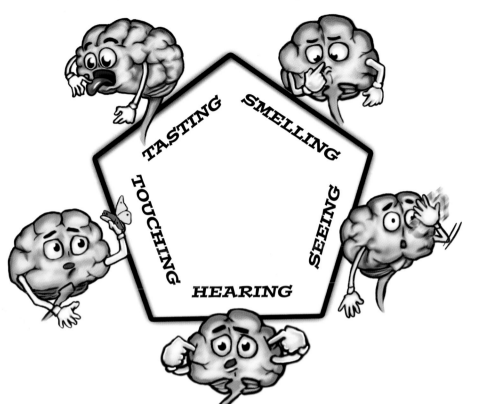

Did you know that injury to Big Boss Brain can also affect the five senses: *hearing*, *seeing*, *smelling*, *tasting*, and *touching*? It can! It can even cause difficulty with balance and headaches. Sometimes Daddy loses his balance walking by himself. He can usually catch himself, but I have to make sure I'm not in his way.

Once, while we were playing, Daddy fell down and his whole body shook. It was very scary. While it was happening, Daddy couldn't talk or move. His body just kept shaking. He was having a *seizure*. Mommy saw what happened and made sure there was nothing sharp or hard around him. She also protected his head with a rolled up blanket so it wouldn't hit the floor. She told me to call 9-1-1. The ambulance came, and the emergency medical technicians (EMTs) helped Daddy. Mommy and one of the EMTs made sure I knew that the seizure was caused by electrical activity in his brain, not anything I did. Seizures can happen after a TBI.

SEIZURE

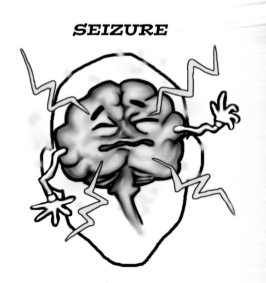

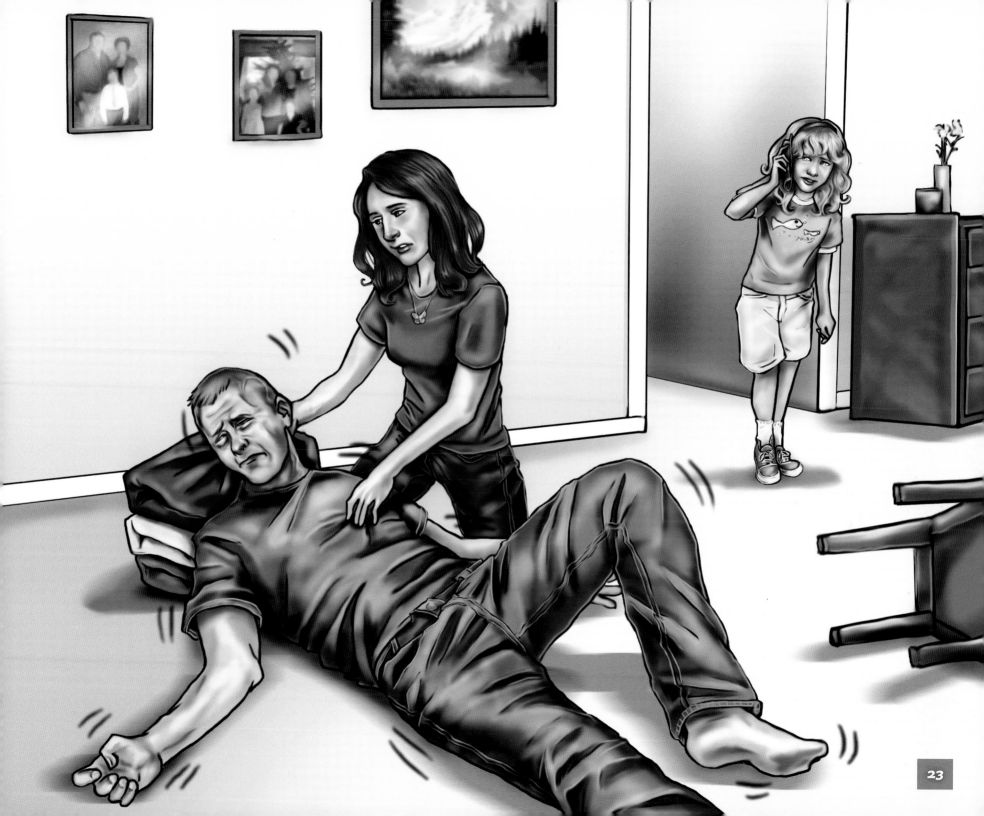

Mommy told me that the doctors would help Daddy. They would give him some medicine to control the seizures. Big seizures like my daddy had that day are called **grand mal** or **generalized seizures**. There are other types of seizures that people with a TBI can also have. These don't always cause a person's body to move. They can simply make a person sit very still, like they are asleep with their eyes open. So don't be scared if this happens. Quickly find an adult and tell them what you saw. Sometimes you can be a helper by being a good observer.

SEIZURE

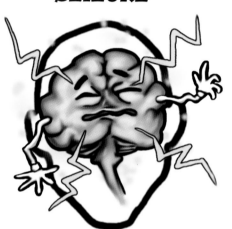

After Daddy's seizure, he had to go back to the hospital for a little while. My mom called my grandma. Grandma came to stay with me and set up some play time with my friends. Mommy said it was important for her to be with Daddy at the hospital. Mostly I understood. I liked spending time with my grandma and my friends. At the same time, I was a little sad and even a little mad. I wondered why it wasn't important for Mommy to be with me. Why couldn't I help Daddy? I was a good helper! I went to my room and hit my pillow. Then I hugged my bear until I was ready to talk to Grandma about what I was feeling.

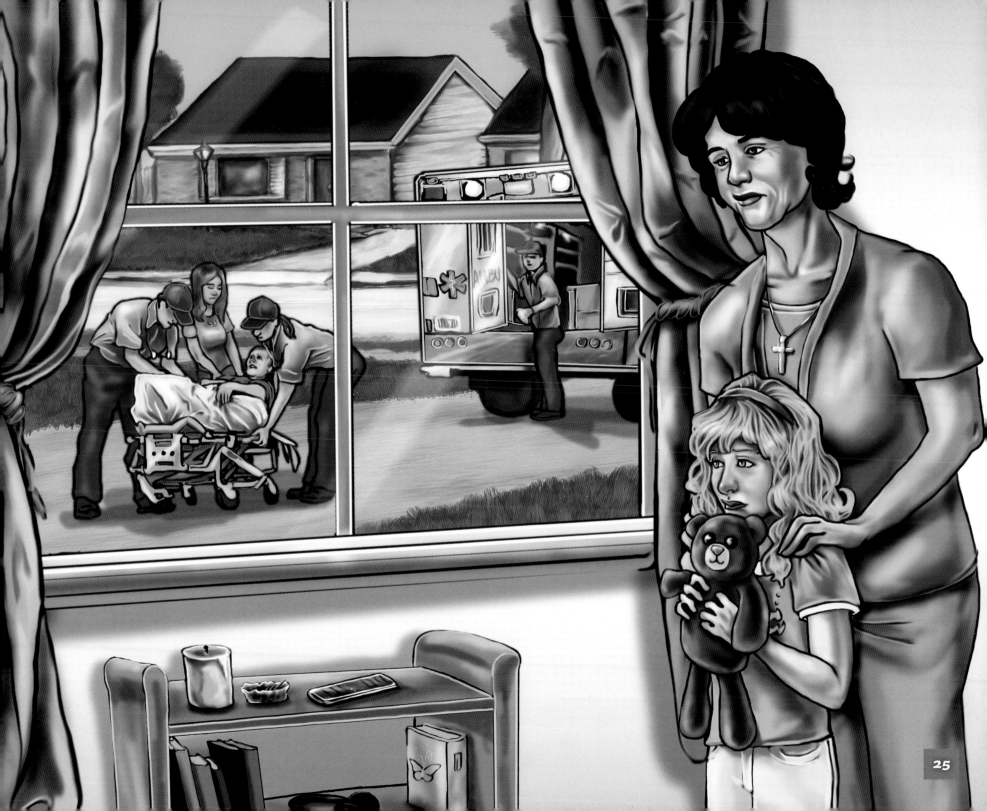

Do you know what? Grandma understood how I felt. She said it was okay for me to have those feelings! The fact that Daddy was hurt and that we had to be apart was not fun or fair. But it didn't change the fact that Mommy and Daddy *loved me* and wanted to be with me. For that time, though, they needed to be where Daddy could get help. Mommy needed to listen to and learn from all that the doctors had to say. That way, when they came back home, they could explain everything to me, my brother, and sister.

At home and at the hospital, Daddy was also feeling sad and mad sometimes—just like me! There were days when he was tired of being injured. He wished it was easier to write or use his right hand. Sometimes his tears or anger came from frustration. Other times, it just came suddenly, out of nowhere. I thought maybe I did something to make him upset. I learned, though, that when a brain is injured, the things in Big Boss Brain that control when we are happy or sad can change too. Sometimes a rush of happiness, sadness, or anger comes without warning or reason.

Doctors called *psychiatrists* and *neuropsychiatrists* can give TBI patients medicines to help even out their *moods*. Neuropsychologists can help TBI patients understand the changes. They can also teach them to better manage feelings and behaviors.

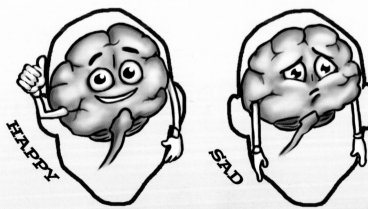

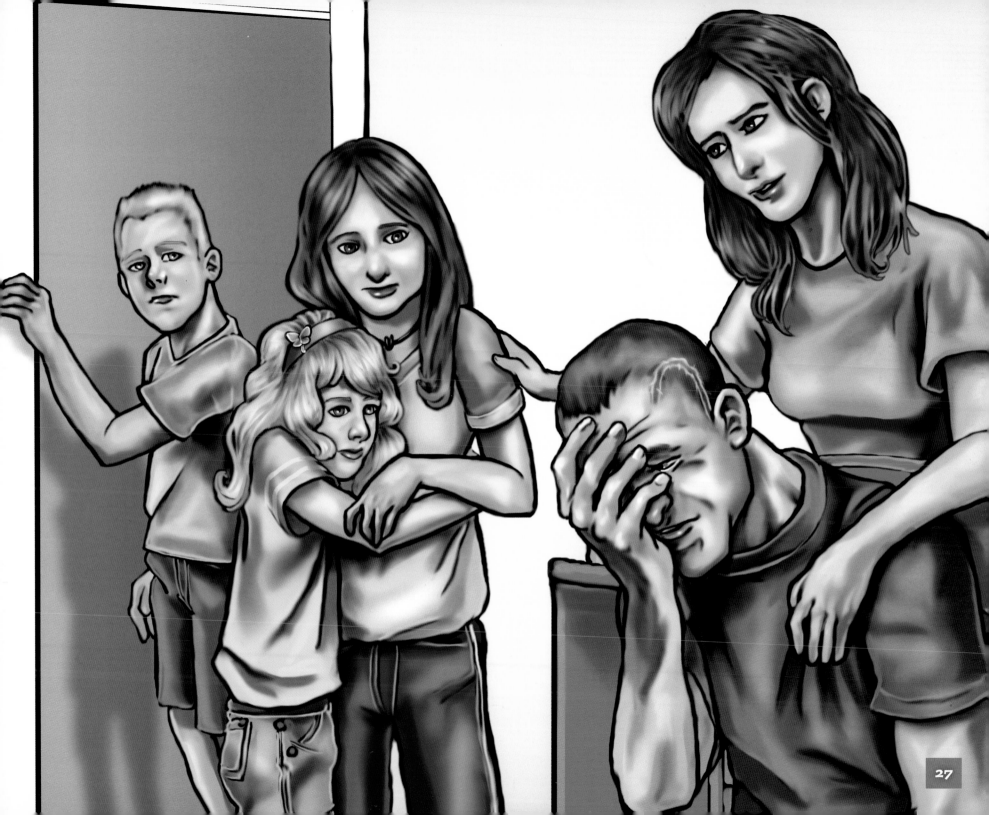

Daddy's changing emotions are some of the **"invisible"** effects of his TBI. We couldn't see them like we could see his right arm not working. But we all felt them just the same. Remember all those other questions swirling in my head: Why did noise bother him so much? Why did he need time alone, and why did he need so much sleep? Why couldn't Daddy go with us to big parties or the amusement park anymore? These are also invisible effects of Big Boss Brain's injury.

After Daddy's TBI, I was told to play quietly a lot more. Daddy needed a lot of sleep. He would take naps during the day, sometimes in his room and other times in his chair in front of the TV. Daddy's

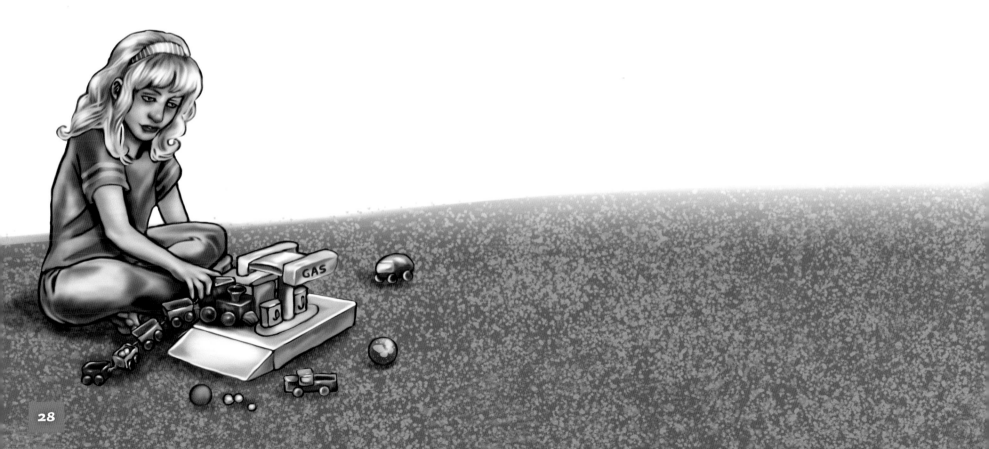

Big Boss Brain was working very hard to get better. It would get tired, and my daddy's body would be tired, too. Daddy told me to picture a **train engine** that couldn't go any farther down the track until it stopped for fuel. Rest was like fuel to Daddy's Big Boss Brain. After some sleep, Daddy was ready to play and work again.

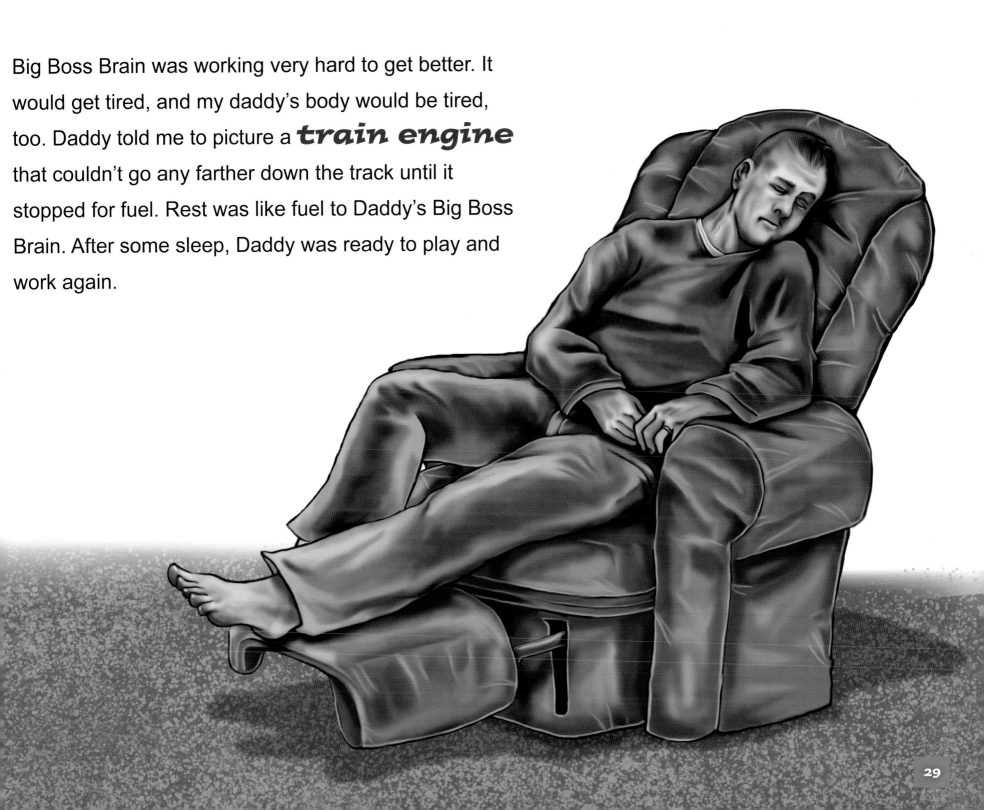

Another reason I had to be quiet was that now too many noises bother Daddy. When Big Boss Brain is *not* hurt, it can focus on one sound and tune out another. Because it **is** hurt, Daddy's Big Boss Brain cannot do that as well. Sounds that used to take turns for his attention now all come rushing in at once.

Remember Daddy's train engine? Imagine that Daddy's Big Boss Brain is the engine. It is chugging along on the main track, carrying the sound of the TV and the dog's barking. On the left, there is a train car coming toward the main track with the voices of my mom and brother talking. On the right, there is another train car carrying a question I have for Daddy, and it's moving toward the track, too.

Normally, crossing bars would stop the train cars on the right and left from entering the main track until it was safe. In the brain, these crossing bars are called *filters*.

When Big Boss Brain is injured, the filters (crossing bars) are broken, so the sounds from the TV, mom talking, and my question all crash into Daddy's brain (the engine) at the same time. What a big mess! It's a mess that Daddy has to work very hard to unscramble. Now I have to help by waiting my turn or making sure the TV is off before asking Daddy a question.

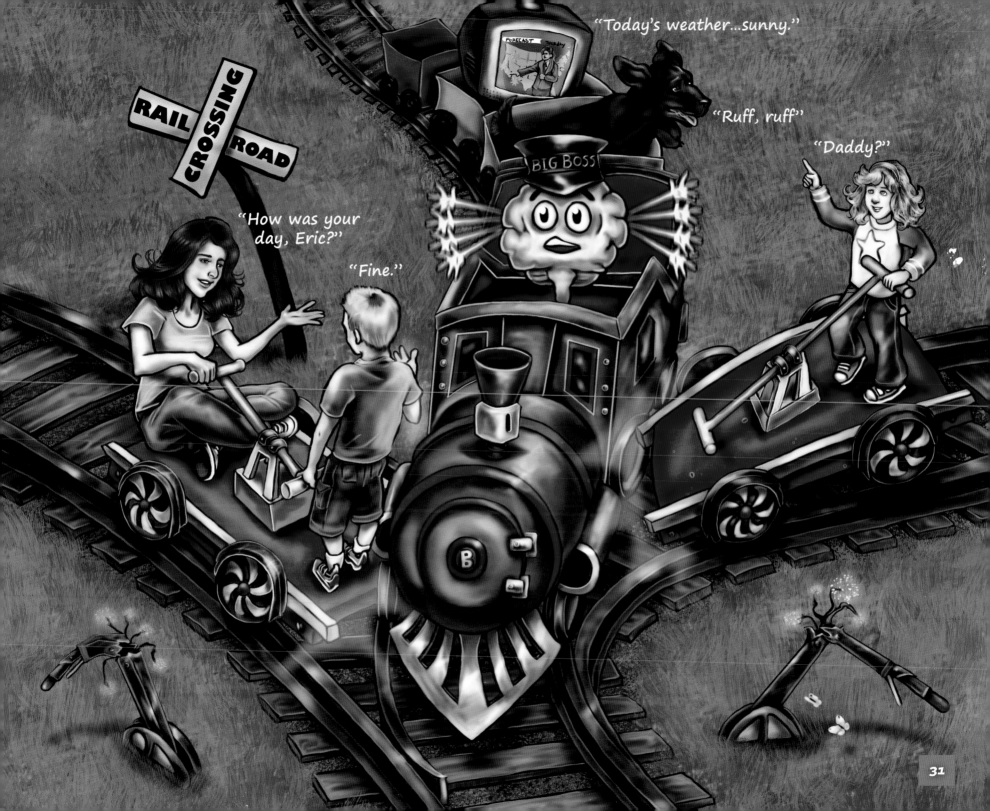

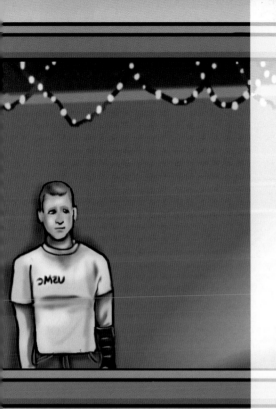

The broken filters in Daddy's Big Boss Brain are also why he has a hard time at big parties or the amusement park. There the voices, sounds of laughter, and even lights can rush in to Daddy's brain all at once. They drain fuel from his Big Boss Brain *"engine."*

At the same time, Daddy's Big Boss Brain works hard to help him walk, watch where he is going, and look around. The fuel empties very quickly. His brain and body become very tired. This is why he often needs time alone. Alone, Daddy can keep one thing on his track and rest Big Boss Brain. He can also stop to get fuel by taking a little nap without stopping our fun at the park or party.

I've learned that we can't always do everything we used to do with Daddy, but we still have special times together. We read together at bedtime. We go on quiet walks with the dog. He comes to my dance performances. Sometimes he stands off to the side alone. Now I know that it's because he's trying to focus on me. He is keeping my train on his track during that time.

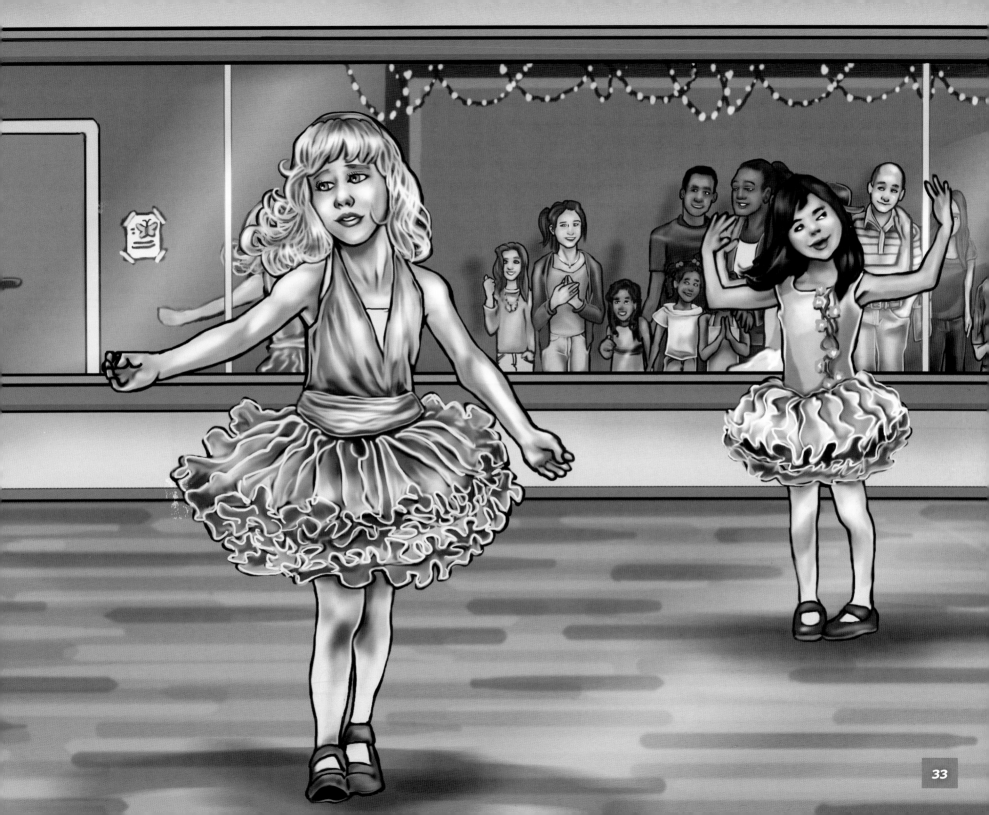

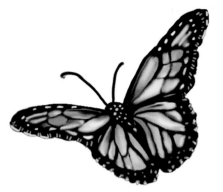

One of the most important things I have learned about TBI is the need for lots of **patience**! That means waiting calmly. It takes time (months, maybe years) for the brain to heal itself. Big Boss Brain may never get completely back to where it started. It also takes Big Boss Brain longer to tell the body what to do. Because of this, I must be more patient when Daddy is answering a question. Sometimes he needs time to think about the answer or turn the other noises off. It is important to wait for him to finish saying what he wants and needs to say. Walking and moving is sometimes slower, too. This is a nice thing on our walks. I get to discover things around me in nature that I might have missed by running or walking too fast.

Life after Daddy's TBI has definitely brought change, but I found out that change is not all bad. I am lucky to still have my daddy here with us. Mommy and Daddy try to keep life at home as routine as possible. Together we're finding what works for us. Along the way, I remember to ask questions. I know that through the ups and downs, whether I'm feeling happy, sad, or mad about our new life after TBI, **I am loved**. And so are you!

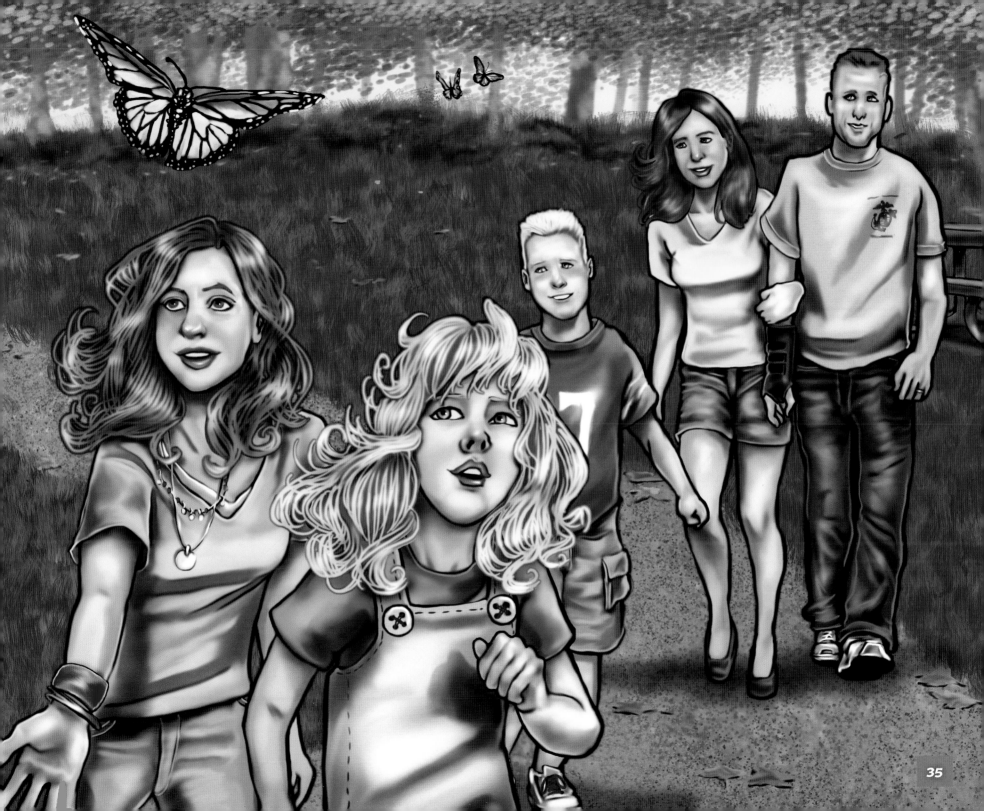

Real Life Stories

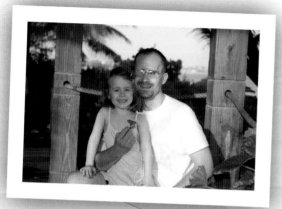

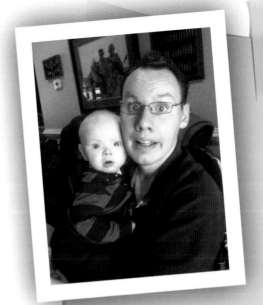

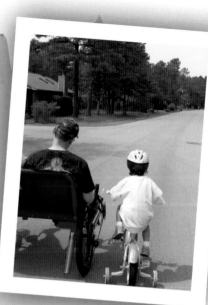

"My daddy got hurt in the Army. He has one eye and hurt his head, but that's okay because he loves me! I like to play with play dough, color, do puzzles, and build things with my daddy!"

—**Alli**, age 4
(*Born 1 month and 1 day
after her dad was injured in Iraq*)
Sun Prairie, WI

"My name is Gracie. My daddy, Eric, was injured in Iraq by a bomb and has a brain injury. I like it when my dad talks to me on his communication device. We like to go to the beach and play in the waves. It is super fun to go paint at Accidental Artist. We also like to ride our bikes together. My little brother, Hunter, is too little to talk, but I can tell he likes Daddy to hold him and push him around in his walker because he smiles!"

—**Gracie**, age 7
(*Age 9 1/2 months when her dad
was wounded and suffered an
anoxic brain injury*) New Bern, NC

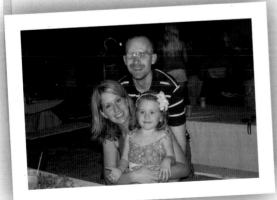

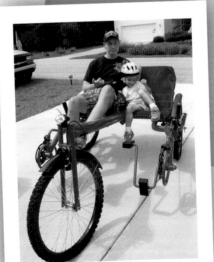

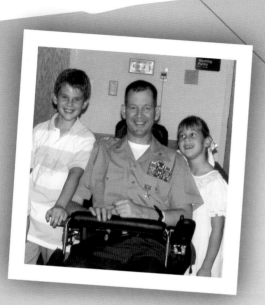

"My dad is doing a lot better now. He can go to movies. He can swim with us. He watches us play outside. I like to do art with my dad and read with him. I always ride on my dad's lap while he drives his wheelchair! My dad still loves us, and we still love him—and that's the best part!"

—**Alaina**, age 7
(*Age 5 when her dad sustained a traumatic brain injury*) Tampa, FL

"Even though my dad got shot in the head, we still do a lot of things you wouldn't imagine we could do. We throw the football, and we play basketball together. We watch a lot of football on TV! He helps me with my homework. We even swim in our pool together (even though he can only move his left arm). I was really sad when my dad got hurt. I am glad he is safe at home now. The best thing about my dad is he's funny. I am proud of my dad for not giving up and always trying harder."

—**Mason**, age 9
(*Age 7 when his dad sustained a traumatic brain injury*) Tampa, FL

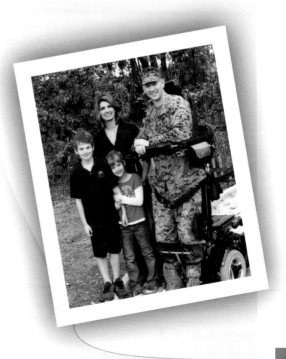

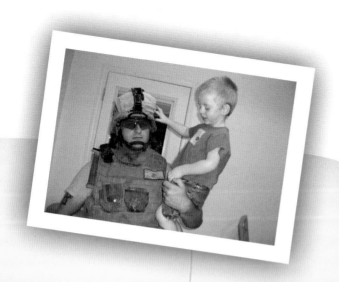

"My daddy is a Marine. He is so cool! He gets to wear a very cool outfit to work. But one day when he was gone, protecting us, the bad people hurt my daddy. They messed up his brain, and now he has seizures. I want to be like my daddy when I grow up, so I can beat up the bad guys who did this to my daddy!"

—**Jase**, age 5

(*Age 2 months when his dad was wounded and 2 ½ when his dad started having seizures*) Jacksonville, NC

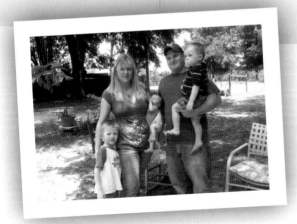

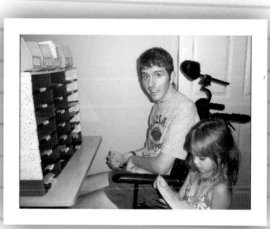

"It's really cool living with my brother. We play with Ben, and I sing to him this song that's a really funny song. Race (age 7) and Reed (age 6), my little brothers, think it's cool living with Ben, too. I like helping to feed him and watching TV with him and playing with him. It's so much fun, but sometimes it's hard not getting to go some places, but we make it work. Race and Reed don't really remember Ben when he played video games and soccer like [them]. Me and Ben always played when I was little, but I still play with him, and it's fun."

—**Jenna**, age 9 (*Age 4 when her brother was hit by a car, crossing a road.*) Blossom, TX

Sammy's Brain Injury

"When I was 11 months old, my mom, my big sister, and I were in a bad car accident. I think my brain injury has affected me because I have to work harder than everyone else. I am always going to a physical therapist, occupational therapist, and all kinds of specialists. I also don't always feel like I fit in, sometimes. I feel like I stand out and that people don't want to hang out with me because of it. But it has also affected me in some good ways. Like I got to meet some really nice people like my counselor and my physical therapist/occupational therapist, who taught me how to walk, and a lot of other cool people who are really nice to me and have helped me to be a stronger person. I think that my brain injury made me have a stronger take on the world and on myself. If it wasn't for my mom and I and all the great specialists trying so hard, I wouldn't have become the person I am today. If we didn't try so hard, my life would be very different. (I know that everybody makes mistakes and that's ok—no one is perfect.) With the right positive attitude and the willingness to accept help, as long as I try my best and I am proud of myself, then move over world—I CAN DO ANYTHING!!!"

—**Samantha**, age 12
(*11 months when she sustained
her brain injury in October 1999*) Beaufort, SC

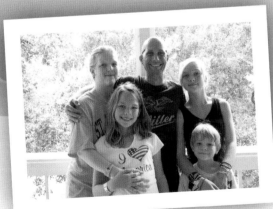

Clues to where the butterflies are: pp. 4-5 coloring page on floor; pp. 6-7 box on dresser; pp. 8-9 Cassidy's belt; pp.10-11 Cassidy's night gown; pp.12-13 SLPs necklace; pp.14-15 Sam's brother's shoulder; pp. 16-17 caseworker's lapel; pp.18-19 refrigerator; pp. 20-21 grass, in front of Jake's dad's hand and the mom's necklace; pp. 24-25 book; pp. 26-27 Cassidy's headband; pp. 28-29 ball; pp. 30-31 near broken crossbar; pp. 22-23 touching brain's hand and girl's necklace; pp. 32-33 on poster on audience (in purple); pp. 34-35 flying overhead

39

The Parts of Big Boss Brain and What They Do

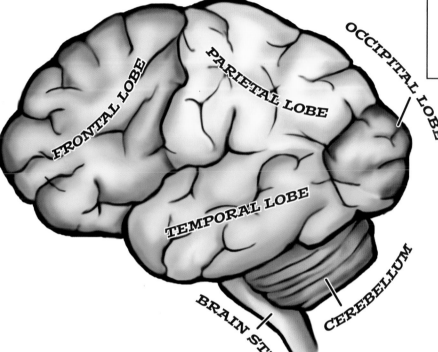

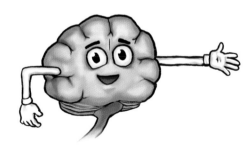

FRONTAL LOBE

- Planning and problem solving
- Emotion
- Personality and behavior
- Movement
- Memory
- Judgment
- Learning
- Thinking
- Smell
- Speech

PARIETAL LOBE

- Touch
- Identification of sizes, shapes, and colors
- Handling of objects
- Combination of senses

OCCIPITAL LOBE

- Sight

CEREBELLUM

- Balance
- Coordination
- Posture

TEMPORAL LOBE

- Memory
- Hearing
- Understanding what we hear and see and making up our replies
- Sorting objects

BRAIN STEM

- Breathing
- Heart rate and blood pressure
- Ability to sleep and alertness
- Sweating
- Temperature
- Swallowing
- Startle reflex
- Balance
- Message path between brain and body